**Patrícia Madruga Rêgo Barros**
**Luciane S. de Lima**

# Depression and Quality of Life in Renal Transplantation

**Patrícia Madruga Rêgo Barros**
**Luciane S. de Lima**


# Depression and Quality of Life in Renal Transplantation

## An analysis of pre- and post-transplant patients


**ScienciaScripts**

This book is a translation from the original published under ISBN 978-613-9-60334-3.

Publisher:
Sciencia Scripts
is a trademark of
Dodo Books Indian Ocean Ltd. and OmniScriptum S.R.L publishing group

120 High Road, East Finchley, London, N2 9ED, United Kingdom
Str. Armeneasca 28/1, office 1, Chisinau MD-2012, Republic of Moldova, Europe
Printed at: see last page
**ISBN: 978-620-7-27310-2**

# SUMMARY

**SUMMARY**

Chronic renal failure (CRF) is a progressive and irreversible deterioration of kidney function, in which the body's ability to maintain metabolic and hydroelephilic balance fails. Its onset is insidious and its main causes are hypertension and diabetes mellitus [12] . The patient with CRF is restricted to two types of treatment: renal replacement therapy or transplantation, the latter being the modality that offers a better quality of life, a possible reduction in the risk of mortality [234] and a lower cost compared to dialysis[2] . The evolution of organ transplantation has represented a major technical and scientific advance, significantly improving the survival of chronic kidney patients and others with chronic diseases. However, important aspects involved in this context, such as emotional and psychosocial aspects, have been neglected[5] . However, these aspects have gained prominence in national and international scientific productions and have had a positive impact on the therapeutic management of patients [5678910] . 'Concern about psychosocial aspects is fundamental to the success of treatment'[6-11] ', as they interfere with the perception and evaluation of the disease, adherence to treatment and the quality of life of patients with chronic renal failure[11] . Considering the importance of the subject for patients with chronic kidney disease who are candidates for kidney transplantation, as well as for post-transplant kidney patients, a study was carried out in 2007 on depression and quality of life in pre- and post-transplant kidney patients followed up at the Kidney Transplant Outpatient Clinic at the Hospital das Clinicas of the Federal University of Pernambuco (HC-UFPE). This research resulted in two articles that make up this master's thesis. The first is a review of the literature on quality of life (QoL) and some historical, ethical, legal and emotional aspects surrounding organ and tissue transplantation, using the Medline, Scielo and Lilacs databases, using the following descriptors: depression, quality of life, organ transplantation, chronic illness. Textbooks and articles cited in the references obtained in the review were also used. The second, in the form of an original article, aimed to analyse the occurrence of depression and quality of life in pre- and post-transplant renal patients followed up at the HC-UFPE Renal Transplant Clinic between July and December 2007.

**Keywords:** depression, quality of life, organ transplant, chronic illness

# REFERENCES

1    Brunner LS, Suddart, DS. New nursing practice. 5ª ed. Rio de Janeiro: Interamericana; 1994.

2    Cunha CB, Leon ACB, Schramm JMA, Carvalho MS, Paulo Júnior RBS, Chain R. Time to transplantation' and survival in patients with chronic renal failure in the State of Rio de Janeiro, Brazil, 1998-2002. Cad saúde pública.2007;23(24):805-13.

3    Castro M, Caiuby AVS, Draibe SA, Canziani MEF.Quality of life of patients with chronic renal failure on haemodialysis assessed using the generic SF-36 instrument.Rev Assoc Med Bras.2003;49(3):245-9.

4    Riella MC. Chronic renal failure: pathophysiology of uremia. In: Riella MC. Principios de nefrologia e distobios hi^oeletroliticos. 3ª ed. Rio de Janeiro: Guanabara Koogan; 1996.cap.36,p.475.

5    Pietrovsk V, Dall'Agnol CM. Significant situations in the space-context of haemodialysis: what do service users say? Rev bras enferm.2006; 59(5):630-5.

6    Contel JOB, Sponholz Jr A, Torrano-Masetti LM,Almeida AC, Oliveira EA, Jesus JS,et al. Psychological and psychiatric aspects of bone marrow transplantation. Medicina (Ribeirão Preto). 2000;33(3):294-311.

7    Mendes AC, Shiratori K. The perceptions of kidney transplant patients. Nursing (São Paulo).2002;5(44):15-22.

8    Virzi A, Signorelli MS, Veroux M, Giammarmsi G, Maugeri S, Nicoletti A, et al. Depression and quality of life in living related renal transplantation.Transplant proc.2007;39(6):1791-3.

9    Shah VS, Ananth A, Sohal GK, Bertges-Yost W, Eshelman A, Parasuraman RK, et al. Quality of life and psychosocial factors in renal transplant recipients. Transplant proc. 2006;38(5): 1283-5.

10   Baines LS, Joseph JT, Jindal RM ve ark.Emotional issues after kidney transplantation: a prospective psychotherapeutic study.Clinfransplant.2002;16(6):450-4.

11   Almeida AM, Meleiro AMAS. Depression and chronic renal failure. J bras nefrol. 2000;22(1):192-200.D

# CHAPTER 1

## REVIEW ARTICLE

**Organ and tissue transplantation: Historical, ethical-legal, emotional aspects and repercussions on quality of life**

**Issues involved in transplantation of organs and tissues: historical, ethical, legal, emotional aspects and its influence in the life quality.**

**Patrícia Madruga Rêgo Barros,** Master's student in Health Sciences at OTPE, specialist in nephrology nursing and nurse at Hospital das Clinicas, Recife-PE, Brazil.

Luciane Soares de Lima, PhD in Pneumological Sciences from UNIFESP/EPM and ProL. Adjunct Professor in the Nursing Department at OTPE.

Address for correspondence:

Patrícia Madruga Rêgo Barcos

Rua Capitão Ponciano, 63 Barco CEP 50780-040 Recife-PE, Brazil.

Tel: (081) 91427665; e - mail: patricia-ma^ga@hotmail.com

**Summary**

Technological advances, which are essential for humanity, have greatly contributed to developments in healthcare. However, humanisation remains a challenge, perhaps because it involves emotional and psychosocial aspects that are fundamental to the success of any type of treatment. Organ and tissue transplants, as an integral part of this technical-scientific evolution, have become a valid option and are often the only viable alternative for the chronically ill. Despite the advances in dialysis treatment, kidney transplantation has been recognised as the best option, with a view to providing a better quality of life for patients with chronic renal failure. However, it is worth emphasising that, like any treatment, transplantation has implications that need to be discussed in order to avoid frustrations and/or emotional and psychological complications for patients who undergo the procedure.

The aim of this article is to present the scientific production on quality of life and some of the historical, ethical, legal and emotional aspects surrounding organ and tissue transplants. Searches were carried out on the Medline, Scielo and Lilacs databases, involving adults, using the following descriptors: depression, quality of life, organ transplantation and chronic illness, as well as textbooks. The scientific production researched revealed two relevant aspects: The first, the significant technological evolution and public policies aimed at organ and tissue transplants in Brazil; The second, however, shows little appreciation of emotional and social aspects, with psychological repercussions and on patients' quality of life. We also observed a disproportion between the number of viable organs for transplantation and the growing waiting list, related to the failure to notify cases of brain death and the approach to requesting donation, resulting in a high number of deaths still on the waiting list. In addition, it was found that the population is unaware of the concept of brain death and is afraid of the organ trade, demonstrating the lack of investment in clarifying these issues and, consequently, the need for educational campaigns to fill this gap.

**Keywords:** depression, quality of life, organ transplant, chronic illness.

## 1.1 Introduction

The development of transplants and their application in the treatment of terminal diseases of certain organs has become one of the most successful themes in the history of medicine. Advances in immunological management, surgical techniques and intensive care, as well as the introduction of more modern immunosuppressive drugs and more efficient preservation solutions, have all contributed to improving the results of transplants[1] .

However, it is important to mention that technical-scientific developments cannot supplant emotional and psychosocial aspects when conducting therapeutic processes[2] . However, this topic has been increasingly valued in scientific research, with a greater number of studies addressing these aspects, which are considered to cause or enhance health problems[3,4,5678]

Ethical aspects are also very important in this context. Transplantation, like any technical-scientific advance that brings significant benefits, also brings ethical issues that should be discussed[9]

.

With regard to patients who have undergone a kidney transplant, in daily practice in a transplant unit, feelings and attitudes such as irritability, anger, guilt, regret, sadness, anxiety are perceived; verbal and physical aggression, hospital avoidance, abandonment of treatment, verbalisation of the wish to die and suicide attempts are also observed. It is believed that these feelings and behaviours may be linked to inadequate management in the preoperative stage of transplants, as well as during hospitalisation, requiring a more humanistic approach to these patients [4,10] .

The decision to have an organ transplant is not an easy one. It involves a series of issues that need to be taken into account, such as socioeconomic, cognitive, cultural, ideological and religious characteristics, as well as the appreciation of each patient's fears, doubts, desires and perspectives, by a multi-professional team that looks at the individual and not just the disease[2,10,11,12] .

All of these factors can have a positive or negative impact on patients' quality of life, given that their meaning is different for each individual^13 , 14-15)

What is worrying is the patient's lack of knowledge or misinformation about the surgery they are about to undergo: the risk of surgery, the clinical and surgical complications in the post-operative period, the possibility of losing the graft, the occasional need for haemodialysis sessions (even after the transplant), dietary restrictions, the number of medications, frequent outpatient monitoring, the wait for care, the need for periodic laboratory tests, the sometimes frequent hospitalisation, as well as the restriction of companions[15] . There are many issues to be assimilated by the patient and their family, and these sudden changes in their lives need to be valued by the healthcare team[10] .

The aim of this article is to present the scientific production on quality of life and the historical, ethical, legal and emotional aspects surrounding organ and tissue transplants.

## 1.2 Method

Medline, Scielo and Lilacs databases were consulted, involving adults, using the following descriptors: depression, quality of life, organ transplantation and chronic illness, as well as textbooks.

## 1.3 Historical aspects

Organ transplantation has been the subject of many attempts over the centuries, but without any chance of success, given the lack of knowledge of the biological phenomena involved in the interaction between the recipient and the graft \.[16]

There are ancient reports on this subject in the literature, dating back to Ayurvedic medicine in India and Greece, but it was during the Second World War that the main biological bases of transplantation were defined, known as the "laws of transplantation". During this period, Peter Medawar and Thomas Gibson carried out experiments with skin transplants on individuals with burns resulting from the war, and described the process of rejection and non-rejection when using grafts from another individual and from the same individual, respectively \.[16]

In 1890, the first bone tissue autotransplant was carried out by the Scotsman Macewen[17] . It wasn't until 1905 that the first experimental organ and tissue transplants began, with the Frenchman Dr Aléxis Carrel as his mentor, who in 1912 was awarded the Nobel Prize for his work[18] \ In 1954, the first successful kidney transplant between univitelline twins was described, carried out by Joseph Murray[17] .

In 1963, the first human liver transplant was attempted in the United States, in Denver, by Thomas Starzl. The patient was a three-year-old child with biliary atresia, who died during surgery due to changes in blood clotting. The second attempt took place months later, performed by the same surgeon. This time on a man, who died twenty days after surgery from thromboembolism[19] .

From 1963 to 1967, several attempts were made in different countries, and in the latter year the first favourable liver transplant result was obtained in a two-year-old girl with cholangiocarcioma. The patient died thirteen months later, however, as a result of metastases from the original disease[19] \ Also in 1967, the first four liver transplant survivors were presented, with the aim of gaining public support to encourage organ donation[19] .

Also in this year, the first heart transplant was described by Bamard and his collaborators at the Groote Schuur Hospital in Cape Town, South Africa, in a patient with left ventricular failure. A year after the first transplants (heart and liver) abroad, the first effective heart transplant took place in Brazil, performed by Professor Zerbini, more precisely on 26 March 1968[18] .

In 1971, the first non-consanguineous inter-vivos kidney transplant was carried out in Brazil, at the Sírio Libanês Hospital in São Paulo[20] .

It is also worth emphasising the importance and history of immunosuppressive drugs in the process of transplant evolution. Over the course of three decades (1955 to 1985), new immunosuppressive drugs were introduced: corticoids, azathioprine, anti-lymphocyte globulin, cyclosporine and OKT3, with the aim of reducing rejection rates and thus increasing transplant survival. In heart transplants, the use of cyclosporine increased patient survival by 75% to 80%[18] .

Also in 1985, the first successful liver transplant in Latin America was performed at the Hospital das Clínicas in São Paulo on a twenty-year-old woman with a primary liver tumour. This patient died thirteen months later as a result of a recurrence of the disease original[19] .

The second group to successfully perform liver transplants in the country was the Children's Institute of the Hospital das Clínicas in São Paulo in 1989. From then on, other states began to carry out the procedure[19] .

The evolution of science has provided the population with significant advances in the field of health. However, political and social aspects surrounding transplants may be hindering the access of a greater number of individuals to the technical and scientific benefits achieved.


## 1.4 Legal and ethical aspects


Brazil is a privileged country when it comes to organ transplant legislation, as it has comprehensive laws that offer safety to both transplanters and users. Until 1997, there was no government policy on transplants in Brazil. Today, it can be said that there is broad and democratic access, regardless of the socioeconomic and cultural level of the patients who need these procedures[16] .

The Unified Health System (SUS) offers full coverage for transplant-related procedures, including post-surgical follow-up, including the supply of immunosuppressants and support medication, for an indefinite period. In the USA, for example, social security and health plans provide partial cover (only for immunosuppressants) and for a limited time after the transplant[16] .

However, there are still some difficulties to be overcome, such as the length of time spent on the transplant waiting list. This may be due to a lack of notification to transplant centres and the failure to use some of the organs donated[16 \ These facts may be related to the failure of health professionals to identify potential donors and to approach them to request donation[20] , as well as the population's lack of knowledge on the subject, religious reasons and the population's insecurity about the effectiveness of public services[21] .

The moment of donation is of fundamental importance, it is a complex stage, as it involves feelings, ethical and legal aspects, and therefore requires a team of professionals who are trained and familiar with the subject in question \(20

With the reduction in the number of viable, deceased donors, the number of living donors increases considerably, in an attempt to meet the repressed demand '[2021] .

However, this is not just the case in Brazil, as countries recognised as having greater technical and financial resources have not yet managed to reduce the waiting list either[16] .

"Transplant systems are currently victims of their own success"[22] . As waiting lists lengthen, in contrast to the availability of organs, which remains stable, there is a high number of deaths in these queues. To try to reverse this situation, the transplant community is reviewing the criteria for donor acceptability, developing new strategies for obtaining organs, accepting cases of procurement after circulatory arrest, marginal donors (donors who fall outside the optimum criteria for donation) and so-called inter-vivos donation .[22]

In terms of Brazilian legislation, the first law to regulate organ transplantation activities was Law No. 5,479, published in August 1968. Until the early 1980s, transplants remained academic in nature, i.e. restricted to clinical research. Only with the emergence of new immunosuppressive therapies could transplantation be considered a real option for patients with chronic renal failure. Outside of universities and with government support, actions to implement, plan and regulate transplants began, due to society's demand for everyone to have the same rights to enjoy this benefit. With the increase in demand, some changes were necessary, including the modernisation of the 1968 law, which did not include, for example, the concept of brain death[16] .

In 1987, the Integrated System for High-Complexity Medical Assistance was set up to plan and regulate dialysis and transplants, and in 1990 it was renamed the Integrated System for High-Complexity Procedures (SIPAC), covering other types of transplant besides kidney transplants. It also incorporated the association of patients and other professionals. This system was abolished in 1992, the year in which the transplant law was amended (Law No. 8,489). This law was only regulated in 1993 by Decree No.[0] 879 of 22 July, which made it compulsory to notify all cases of brain death on an emergency basis[16].

Since then, any public or private service that diagnoses brain-dead patients must notify the Organ Notification, Training and Distribution Centres (CNCDO) so that they can be included as potential organ donors. In addition, for an organ to be used for transplantation, family members must agree to the donation \.[19]

Once the diagnosis of brain death has been established, professionals are free to act in front of family members or legal donors and proceed to request the organs, followed by the signature of the person responsible and two witnesses (not part of the transplant or neurological recovery team) on the donation form[20].

In 1997, through Resolution No. 1,480 of the Federal Council of Medicine, paediatric patients were included in the criteria for brain death. In the same year, Law No. 9,434 was passed, instituting presumed organ donation in the country by issuing civil identity cards. This law stipulated that all people should state on their identity card and national driving licence whether or not they wished to donate their organs in the event of death \.[16]

This law had a major impact on the population, prompting a mobilisation of the medical profession, patients and representative bodies, which led to the enactment of Law No. 10.211, which put an end to presumed donation[16].

In 1997, the National Transplant System (SNT) was set up to develop the "process of capturing and distributing tissues, organs and parts removed from the human body for therapeutic purposes"[1] -[16] \ Months later, the State Transplant System was set up, responsible for creating technical registers for candidates to receive cadaver organs, the regionalisation of the kidney and liver registers, the centralisation and distribution of the organs procured, adopting the criteria determined by legislation, including Human Lymphocyte Antigen (HLA) compatibility for kidney transplants, and also the creation of organ procurement organisations to decentralise the search for and preparation of donors[16].

The years 1997 and 1998 saw a great deal of movement in the area of transplants, as there was greater participation from society, with the Brazilian Organ Transplant Association standing out \.[1]

In 1998, a number of Ministerial Decrees were instituted relating to transplant management;

Decree No. 3,407 approved the technical regulations on transplant activities and the National Transplant Coordination. Ordinance No. 3,410 established the tables for payment of donor search and preparation, implantation surgeries for the removed organs and post-transplant outpatient follow-up, corresponding to one of the most important steps in the history of transplants, since, in Brazil, until then there had only been coverage for transplants with living donors[1] .

Following the establishment of a transplant policy in the country, the number of kidney and liver transplants increased even more, with 3,362 kidney transplants carried out in 2005, making the country third in the world for this procedure (behind only the USA and China). Liver transplants rose from 1.4 per million population (pmp) in 1997 to 5.6 pmp in 2005, totalling 956 transplants. Pancreas transplants have also increased significantly since 2000. °In 2006, Brazil was in 5th place in South America in terms of transplants, with 6.0 pmp, behind Uruguay with 25.2 pmp, Argentina with 11.68 pmp, Chile with 10.1 pmp and Colombia with 9.9 pmp[21] .

Bioethics is closely linked to the issue of transplants. Its field of action and reflection emphasises research of a psychosociological nature, as well as research related to intensive care medicine. In the latter, among other things, issues arising from substitute medicine, such as transplants, stand out. In this sense, ethical conflicts have been highlighted, such as the definition of brain death^.

The need to define brain death arose with the development of intensive care units and respirators capable of sustaining organisms with this diagnosis for hours and even days, as well as the development of transplant techniques. As there is no unanimity on this definition, speculation has arisen, making it difficult to reach a political consensus. Pluralism has been advocated in order to allow for variations in definitions based on individual and group preferences as a solution to this impasse[9] .

However, it should be emphasised that this occurrence of varied definitions can lead to serious problems, because even in pluralistic societies there is a need to define death. The problems raised by the definition of death are complex, as they are related to various factors, including beliefs, scientific and philosophical positions[9] .

The importance of this topic is related to one of the most complex ethical aspects inherent in organ transplants. Many patients report their doubts about the uncertainty surrounding the death of the donor of the organ they received, which generates anxiety, fear and insecurity about whether or not to have the transplant. The fact that the patient knows that they have an organ that doesn't belong to them and that a person had to die so that they could live seems to increase the affective need '[923)

.

According to article 4° of Resolution No. 1480/97 of the Federal Council of Medicine:

It is therefore essential to clarify the meaning of brain death to the public, presenting all the diagnostic criteria in an accessible way, with scientific rigour, so as not to raise doubts.

Another pertinent discussion in the field of bioethics concerns the principles of autonomy, beneficence, non-maleficence and justice. These principles should be considered the basis of professional ethics in the health area[25] . Due to the closer relationship with the subject, we have chosen to contextualise only the first principle.

Autonomy is "the principle that concerns the professional's duty to give all necessary information and the patient's right to receive clear information adapted to their understanding, so that they can decide about their situation"[25 ,26] .

The right to free and informed consent comprises: "The right to give consent, to participate in treatment without coercion, without being deceived and with competence; as well as the right to withdraw from treatment at any time."[9 ,26] .

From this perspective, an important aspect to consider is the emotional aspect, which is at the heart of the issue of informed consent. As individuals are both rational and emotional, they may suffer external influences and even unconscious motivations when making decisions[9] .

Therefore, the following questions are valid: does the moment when the patient asks for the graft to be removed (due to clinical or surgical complications) and expresses the desire to return to the "haemodialysis machine" correspond to a moment of fragility? The pain, the use of immunosuppressants, the prolonged period of hospitalisation, the frustration of his prospects, the concern for his family at home, the fear of a major complication leading to his death? Who can know for sure if the request to remove the organ isn't a cry for help?

The conclusion that can be drawn from this problem is that the individual's decision should be respected, but that they should be given full information about the implications of their actions, guaranteeing their freedom and dignity[9] .


Another ethical aspect that must be considered in the context of organ and tissue transplants is the trade in organs. The possibility of trading organs from a living donor who is not related to the recipient is a question that is pertinent to bioethics and the law. Law No. 9.434, of 4 February 1997, allowed the donation of organs while alive by non-relatives, provided they were legally capable and did not compromise the donor's health; however, even though it was expressly provided for, free donation could still give rise to the sale of organs[27] .

Then, on 23 March 2001, Law No. 10,211 was enacted:

The intention to buy and sell can be masked by altruistic claims of helping others, taking into account the vulnerable condition of the donor, as well as that of the recipient, due to the imminence of death[27] .

## 1.5 Quality of life and emotional aspects

Quality of Life is defined as: "an individual's perception of their position in life, in the context of the culture and value system in which they live and in relation to their goals, expectations, standards and concerns"[13] .

Quality of Life covers domains of functioning such as psychological conditions and well-being, social interactions, economic and/or vocational conditions or factors, and religious and/or spiritual conditions[13] . Quality of Life is assessed through the individual's perception of each of these areas '[1328] .

With regard to patients with chronic renal failure (CRF), the use of technological resources for therapeutic purposes may not be enough to improve their quality of life[29] . The patient becomes dependent on dialysis treatment, which causes a rise in anxiety levels, among other psychological changes, resulting in a drop in productivity and family income, a reduction in social activities and job opportunities, a limitation in life expectancy and a loss of self-esteem '[1530] ; physical or mental sequelae are often evident .[29]

Transplantation then appears as the "key" to solving all the problems of chronic kidney disease, an alternative for improving the quality of life of this clientele^ '[1531] -*. It's a technically complex and psychologically difficult decision '[1532] .

Health professionals are responsible for assessing the patient's general condition, the risks that may occur and the possible improvements for them, since they are facing a major decision that concerns their personal identity, their life and their death[32] .

However, the prolonged wait for a transplant can lead to other complications for the patient, making them high risk and consequently increasing the number of deaths. Patients experience a great deal of anxiety and emotional deprivation related to their difficult journey. They are also affected by fear, related to the uncertainty of the disease's evolution, the possibility of rejection, the need for medication for the rest of their lives, the uncertain waiting period for the transplant, the impossibility of carrying out the surgical procedure and the delay in discharge due to complications '[1123] .

The prospect of improving quality of life through transplantation can be frustrated by problems that occur after surgery, such as graft rejection or adverse effects caused by immunosuppressants '[1533] .

However, for many patients with chronic renal failure, transplantation is still the best option, as it offers the best chance of survival and rehabilitation, at a lower social cost than dialysis ' '(13134) . Examples include the majority of chronic uremics, patients with end-stage renal failure ' '(143435) , patients with end-stage heart disease, liver disease or lung disease, and for the latter, transplantation is even more valuable, as it is the only therapeutic option capable of preventing death within a few months, offering the prospect of a new life '(134) .

The long period of dialysis treatment leads to a number of problems, such as bone complications (osteodystrophy due to secondary hyperparathyroidism), cardiovascular complications (left ventricular hypertrophy, vascular calcification), cerebral complications (advanced arteriosclerosis), and the chance of death among haemodialysis patients is 20 times higher than in the general population '(2835) .

Even in the face of so many complications related to haemodialysis, it is worth pointing out that kidney transplantation should not be considered as the salvation for all the problems of chronic kidney disease patients; it should be considered as another treatment option, which may present complications, like any other intervention. However, understanding aspects associated with quality of life and coping strategies used by patients undergoing kidney transplantation can help in the development of preventive and intervention programmes suited to the needs of these patients '(1315) .

In a study on the psychological and psychiatric aspects of bone marrow transplantation (BMT), it was mentioned that:

> The intensity and complexity involved in BMT, at its various levels, produce profound psychological effects on the patient, their family and their professional team and emphasise that ignoring this reality and reducing the problems of BMT to their purely technical aspects can have catastrophic consequences for the patient and their family and threaten the survival of the team \.(4

In order to reduce alterations such as those described above, preoperative psychological care is essential^ '011-36 \ This preparation helps to identify high-risk patients who need rigorous psychological care, and even to restrict or contraindicate transplantation as a treatment(36) .

Depressive syndrome is common in almost all chronic diseases and is responsible for poor adherence to proposed treatments, poor quality of life and higher morbidity and mortality among patients(37) .

This disorder is the most common psychological complication in dialysis patients and is a response to a real, threatened or imagined loss. The psychological manifestations observed in these patients are: persistent depressed mood, impaired self-image and pessimistic feelings. Physiological complaints include sleep disturbance, changes in appetite and weight, dryness of the oral mucosa, constipation and decreased sexual interest '(3839 \ It should also be noted that symptoms of depression should be analysed very carefully, as they can be confused with symptoms of uremia \[39]

Depression affects patients both pre- and post-transplant. In general, there are four main types of depression: Adjustment Disorder with Depressed Mood, Depressive Disorders, Bipolar Disorders and Mood Disorders Due to Illness or Drug[40] . The first and last are emphasised due to their greater identification with the characteristics presented by chronic and transplanted patients.

In Adjustment Disorder with Depressed Mood, depression can be related to a stressor. The patient may mention the death of a loved one, a divorce, a financial setback or the loss of an established role in society that made them feel needed in some activity, and this loss results in a feeling of guilt. The disorder occurs within three months of the event and leads to changes in social activity.

Symptoms range from mild sadness, anxiety, irritability, worry, lack of concentration, discouragement and somatic complaints. Mood Disorder Due to Illness or Drugs mainly affects patients with chronic illnesses. Conditions such as rheumatoid arthritis, multiple sclerosis, chronic heart disease and others can lead to depressive disorders[40] .

With regard to the complications of depression, the longer it lasts, the more entrenched it becomes. Suicide is mentioned as the most significant complication. Patients with cancer, respiratory diseases, acquired immunodeficiency syndrome and those on haemodialysis have higher suicide rates[40] . As for kidney transplant patients, depression is inversely related to graft survival time, but it may be the consequence of graft loss rather than its cause .[5]

In Brazil, the prevalence of depression is between 5% and 25% in kidney transplant patients. The consequences of depression have a significant impact on quality of life, suicide rates, adherence to treatment and mortality[30] .

## 1.6 Final considerations

Two main aspects should be emphasised in relation to transplants: the significant technological evolution and public policies aimed at organ and tissue transplants in Brazil, as well as the evidence that little value is placed on emotional and social aspects, with beneficial psychological repercussions and on patients' quality of life.

On the other hand, the literature describes that there is still a lack of preparation on the part of health professionals when it comes to diagnosing brain death and identifying a possible donor, as well as when it comes to reporting cases to transplant centres and approaching family members when they request a donation, and cites an increase in the number of deaths on waiting lists as a consequence.

It is a priority to have trained multi-professional teams, fully capable of collaborating, in their specific areas, in the organ donation process and in preparing the patient for transplantation.

**References**

1  Garcia VD, Abbud-Filho M, Campos HH, Pestana JOM. Transplant policy in Brazil In: Garcia VD, Abbud Filho M, Neumann J, Pestana JOM. Organ and tissue transplantation. São Paulo: Segmento Farma Editora; 2006. p. 43-9.

2  Pietrovsk V, DalíAgnol CM. Significant situations in the space-context of haemodialysis: what do service users say? Rev bras enferm. 2006; 59(5):630-5.

3  Brandão de Carvalho Lira AL, Cavalcante Guedes MV, Oliveira Lopes MV. Adolescente renal crónico: alteraciones físicas, sociales y emocionales pos-trasplante. Rev Soc Esp Enferm Nefrol. 2005;8(4):12-6.

4  Contei JOB, Sponholz Jr A, Torrano-Massetti LM, Almeida AC, Oliveira EA, Jesus JS, et al. Psychological and psychiatric aspects of bone marrow transplantation. Medicina, Ribeirão Preto. 2000;33(3):294-311.

5  Akman B, Ozdemir FN, Sezer S, Micozkadioglu H, Haberal M. Depression levels before and after renal transplantation. Transplant proc. 2004;36(l): 111-3.

6  Zimmermann PR, Carvalho JO, Mari JJ. Impact of depression and other psychosocial factors on the prognosis of chronic renal patients. Rev psiquiatr Rio Gd Sul. 2004; 26(3):312-8.

7  Amâncio JS, Borges MP, Oliveira A, Magalhães EF, Oliveira LHS, Bemardes RC. Evaluation of the quality of life and complaints of chronic renal patients undergoing haemodialysis. In: Proceedings of the XI Latin American Scientific Initiation Meeting, VII Latin American Postgraduate Meeting - Vale do Paraíba University, I High School Scientific Initiation Meeting; 2007; São José dos Campos. São José dos Campos: Universidade do Vale do Paraíba; 2007. p. 2011-4.

8  Virzi A, Signorelli MS, VerouxM, Giammarresi G, Maugeri S, Nicoletti A, et al. Depression and quality of life in living related renal transplantation. Transplant proc. 2007;39(6): 1791-3.

9  Torres WC. Bioethics and health psychology: reflections on questions of life and death. Psicol reflex crit. 2003;16(3):475- 82.

10  Castro EK. The chronic kidney patient and organ transplantation in Brazil: psychosocial aspects. Rev SBPH. 2005;8(l):l-14.

11  Martins PD, Sankarankutty AK, Silva OC, Gorayeb R. Psychic distress in patients listed for liver transplantation. Acta cir bras. 2006;21 Suppl 1: 40-3

12  Pereira E, Menegatti C, Percegona L, Aita CA, Riella MC. Psychological aspects of diabetic patients who are candidates for pancreatic islet transplantation. Arq bras psicol [journal on the

Internet]. 2007 Aug 22 [access in 2008 Sep 22]. Available at: http: // seer.psicologia.ufij .br/seer/lab 19/oj s/viewarticle.php?id=23.

13  Ravagnani LMB, Domingos NAM, Miyazaki MCOS. Quality of life and coping strategies in patients undergoing kidney transplantation. Estud psicol. (Natal). 2007; 12 (2): 177-84.

14  Pereira LC, Chang J, Fadil-Romão MA, Abensur H, Araújo MRT, Noronha IL, et al. Health-related quality of life in renal transplant patients. J bras nefrol. 2003;25(l):10-6.

15  Mendes AC, Shiratori K. The perceptions of kidney transplant patients. Nursing (São Paulo). 2002;5(44): 15-22.

16  Manfro RC, Noronha IL, Silva Filho AP, editors. Manual of kidney transplantation. Iª ed. São Paulo: Manole; 2004.

17  Barcellos FC. Intention to donate organs in an adult population [dissertation on the Internet]. Pelotas: Federal University of Pelotas, Faculty of Medicine; 2003 [2008 Oct 24]. Available from: http://www.abto.org.br/profissionais

18  Silva PR. Heart and cardiopulmonary transplantation: 100 years of history and 40 years of existence. Rev Bras Cir Cardiovasc. 2008;23(l): 145-52.

19  Mies S. Liver transplantation. AMB rev. Assoe. Med. Bras. 1998;44(2): 127-34.

20  Cavalcanti FCB, Paula FJ. Family members' approach to cadaver organ donation In: Cruz J, Barros RT, organisers. Current events in nephrology. São Paulo: Sarvier;1996. v. 4, p. 276-9.
21  Rosa TN. Bioethics and cadaver donor confidentiality in kidney transplants dissertation on the Internet]. Brasília: Federal University of Brasília, Faculty of Health Sciences; 2007      [ 2008Sept23      ].      Disponívelem : http://bdtd.bce.unb.br/tedesimplificado/tde_arquivos/6/TDE-2008-04-11T152850Z-2525/Publico/Dissertacao_Telma%20Rosa.pdf

22  D'Império F. Brain death, organ donor care and lung transplantation. Rev. bras. ter. intensiva [journal on the Internet]. 2007 Jan-Mar [access in 2008 Nov 30]; 19(l):[about 10p. ]. Available at: http://www.scielo.br/scielo.php?script=sci_arttext&pid=S0103-507X2007000100010&lng=en. doí: 10.1590/S0103-507X2007000100010

23  Massarollo MC, Kurcgant P. The experience of nurses in the liver transplant programme of a public hospital. Rev latinoam enferm. 2000;8(4):66-72.

24  Queiroz, VS. Reflexões acerca da equação da anencefalia à morte encefálica como justificativa para a interrupção da gestação de fetos anencefállicos . Jus Navigandi, 3 Aug. 2005 9(760).

25  Junges JR. Bioethics: hermeneutics and casuistry. São Paulo: Loyola; 2006.

26  Fabbro, L. Legal limitations to patient autonomy. Rev. Bioét [journal on the Internet]. 1999 [access in 2007 Aug 23]; 7(l):[about 5 p.]. Available at: http://www.cremeb.cfm.org.br/revista/indlv7.htm

27  Passarinho LEV, Gonçalves MP, Garrafa V. Bioethical study of kidney transplants with non-parent living donors in Brazil: the ineffectiveness of legislation in preventing organ trade. AMB rev. Assoe. Med. Bras [periodical on the Internet]. 2003 [access in 2008 Nov 30]; 49(4):[about 8p.                                      ].          Available at: http://www.scielo.br/scielo.php?script=sci_arttext&pid=S0104- 42302003000400028&lng=en. doi: 10.1590/S0104-42302003000400028.

28  Amato MS, Amato Neto V, Uip DE. Evaluation of the quality of life of patients with Chagas' disease undergoing heart transplantation. Rev Soc Bras Med Trop. 1997;30(2): 159-60.

29  Zanei SS. Analysis of the WHOQOL-BREF and SF-36 quality of life assessment instruments: reliability, validity and agreement among intensive care unit patients and their families [thesis]. São Paulo: University of São Paulo; 2006.
30  Almeida AM, Meleiro AMAS. Depression and chronic renal failure. J bras nefrol. 2000; 22(1): 192-200.

31  Cunha CB, Leon ACB, Schramm JMA, Carvalho MS, Paulo Júnior RBS, Chain R. Time to transplantation and survival in patients with chronic renal failure in the State of Rio de Janeiro, Brazil, 1998-2002. Cad saúde pública. 2007;23(24);805-13.

32  Steiner P, Vieira MCR. Organ donation: the law, the market and families. Tempo Soc [periodical on the Internet]. 2004 Nov [accessed 2008 Nov 30]; 16(2):[about 22 p.]. Available at: http://www.scielo.br/scielo.php?script=sci_arttext&pid=S0103- 20702004000200005&lng=en&nrm=iso doi: 10.1590/S0103-20702004000200005.

33  Bittencourt ZZLC, Alves Filho G, Mazzali M, Santos NR. Quality of life in kidney transplant patients: importance of the functioning graft. Rev Saúde Pública. 2004; 38(5):732-4.

34  Garcia VD. Por uma política de transplantes no Brasil, Office Editora e Publicidade Ltda, São Paulo (2000).

35  Santos PR, Pontes LR Sansigolo K. Change in quality of life in patients with end-stage renal failure during 12-month follow-up. AMB rev. Assoe. Med. Bras [periodical on the Internet]. 2007 Aug [access in 2008 Nov 29]; 53(4):[about 5 p.]. Available at:

http://www.scielo.br/scielo.php?script=sci_arttext&pid=S0104-  42302007000400018&lng=en. doi: 10.1590/S0104-42302007000400018

36  Silva, RMG. The importance of psychological aspects in the indication for kidney transplantation and its bioethical implications [dissertation]. Joinville (SC): Universidade da Região de Joinville; 2003.

37  Teng CT, Humes EC, Demetrio FN. Depression and clinical comorbidities. Rev psiquiatr clín (São Paulo). 2005;32(3): 149-59.

38  Kimmel PL, Peterson RA, Weihs KL, Simmens SJ, Alleyne S, Cruz I, et al. Multiple measurements of depression predict mortality in a longitudinal study of chronic haemodialysis outpatients. Kidney Int. 2000;57(5):2093-8.

39  Daugirdas JT, Blake PG, Ing TS, editors. Manual of dialysis. 3ª ed. Rio de Janeiro: Medsi, 2003.
40  Tiemey LM Jr, McPhee SJ, Papadakis MA. Lange diagnosis and treatment. São Paulo: Atheneu; 1998.

# CHAPTER 2

## ORIGINAL ARTICLE

**Depression and quality of life in patients before and after kidney transplantation***

**Depression and quality of life in patients with pre and post kidney transplantation**

**Patrícia Madruga Rêgo Barros,** Master's student in Health Sciences at UFPE, specialist in nephrology nursing and nurse at Hospital das Clínicas, Recife-PE, Brazil.
Luciane Soares de Lima, PhD in Pneumological Sciences from UNIFESP/EPM and Prof[1] . Adjunct Professor in the Nursing Department at UFPE.

*Study carried out at the Renal Transplant Ambulatory of the Hospital das Clínicas of the Federal University of Pernambuco, Recife, Brazil.

Address for correspondence:
Patrícia Madruga Rêgo Barros
Rua Capitão Ponciano, 63 CEP 50780-40 - Recife, PE, - Brazil
e-mail: patricia-madruga@hotmail.com

### Summary

**Objective: To** analyse the occurrence of depression and quality of life in pre- and post-transplant renal patients followed up at the Renal Transplant Outpatient Clinic at the Hospital das Clínicas of the Federal University of Pernambuco (HC-UFPE). **Method: A** descriptive exploratory study with a quantitative cross-sectional approach, carried out between July and December 2007. Three instruments were used to collect data: a questionnaire to characterise the sample, the Beck Depression Inventory (BDI) and the SF-36 questionnaire to assess quality of life. The sample consisted of two groups, one of pre-renal transplant patients (59 patients) and the other of renal transplant patients (63 patients), totalling 122 patients. The inclusion criteria were: being over 18 years old and between 6 months and 2 years after transplantation. The exclusion criterion was having a previous diagnosis of psychiatric illness. **Results:** The average age of the pre-transplant patients was 47 years, 57.6% of whom were male, and that of the transplant patients was 39 years, 55.6% of whom were male. The average time on dialysis in the first group was 3 years and 3 months and in the second group it was 6 years and 8 months. The average transplant time was 1 year and 3 months. The majority of patients in both groups were not depressed, corresponding to 88.9% of transplant patients and 79.6% of pre-transplant patients. Among those with some degree of depression, there was no significant difference between being pre-transplant or having already undergone transplantation (p = 0.470). The length of time since kidney transplantation and dialysis treatment also showed no relationship with the levels of depression found (p = 0.547 and p = 0.089) respectively. Quality of life was higher in transplanted patients than in those awaiting the procedure. The domains of the SF-36 questionnaire that determined the best quality of life in transplant patients were functional capacity (p = 0.001), pain (p = 0.027), general state of health (p = 0.049) and vitality (p = 0.000). **Conclusion:** This study showed a low occurrence of depression in both pre- and post-renal transplant patients. Quality of life was higher in the transplant group.

**Keywords:** Depression, quality of life, organ transplantation, chronic illness.

## 2.1 Introduction

Chronic renal failure (CRF) can be conceptualised as a slow and progressive loss of kidney function, resulting in abnormalities of the internal environment such as azotemia, anaemia, metabolic acidosis, hyperphosphataemia, hypercalcaemia and hyponatremia. Elevated serum levels, especially of urea, and creatinine clearance of less than 10 ml/min characterise uremic syndrome, the signs and symptoms of which particularly involve the gastrointestinal, nervous and cardiopulmonary tracts. Patients may experience weakness, nausea, vomiting, anorexia, gastrointestinal bleeding, paresthesia, hypertension, irritability, anxiety, depression, among others[1] .

As it is a progressive disease, its development is not the same for all individuals, varying according to its underlying causes, the rate of protein excretion in the urine and the degree of hypertension of each patient[2] .

CRF is divided into stages according to the patient's kidney function. Initially, there is no kidney damage or altered kidney function. Gradually, the kidneys reduce their filtration rate, serum urea and creatinine changes occur and signs and symptoms associated with the underlying cause appear. Finally, the kidneys lose control of the internal environment, requiring renal replacement therapy (RRT)[3] .

Renal replacement therapy aims to maintain the patient in suitable conditions from a metabolic and clinical point of view, as well as adapting to treatment. However, when it comes to dialysis, total rehabilitation is not achieved, unlike transplants which successfully rehabilitate subjectively and objectively, and with excellent cost/benefit ratio[4] .

Advances in dialysis technology have contributed substantially to increasing the survival of patients with CRF [56] . However, remaining on dialysis treatment for an indefinite period of time can interfere with their quality of life .[5]

Studies show a better quality of life after transplantation '[78] , due to the possibility of returning to normal activities, however, transplantation may be related to unsatisfactory scores among those who have had acute rejection, or adverse effects from the use of immunosuppressants[7] .

Currently, quality of life is defined according to the area of application, encompassing two trends: the first presents a generic concept, which emphasises aspects related to the degree of satisfaction found in family, affective, social and environmental life, correlating with the standard that society considers to be comfort and well-being. The second trend is related to health and considers the influence of illnesses and their treatments on patients' quality of life[9] .

Health-related quality of life is conditioned by the experiences of each patient, i.e. how the effects of the disease and its treatment affect the daily life and satisfaction of each individual^' '101 r) .

Concern about psychosocial aspects is fundamental to the success of treatment[1213] , as these directly interfere with the perception and evaluation of the disease, adherence to treatment and the quality of life of patients with CRF[13] .

Depression is considered the most common psychological complication in dialysis patients. Among the most common psychological manifestations in this clientele are: persistent depressed mood, impaired self-image and feelings of pessimism. Physiological complaints include: changes in appetite and weight, sleep disturbances and reduced sexual interest[14] . Candidates for kidney transplantation often experience psychological changes and depression is one of these[15] .

Transplant patients may experience loss of interest in almost all activities, as well as reduced appetite, sleep disturbances, decreased energy, feelings of guilt or worthlessness and impaired thinking. There may often be thoughts of death, suicidal ideation or attempted suicide, which are more common in cases of organ rejection and return to dialysis \.[1516

The above shows the importance of emotional aspects and quality of life in monitoring patients with CRF who are waiting for an organ in the pre-transplant queue, as well as those who have already undergone the procedure.

The aim of the study was to analyse the occurrence of depression and quality of life in pre- and post-transplant kidney patients followed up at the Renal Transplant Outpatient Clinic at the Hospital das Clínicas (HC) of the Federal University of Pernambuco (UFPE).

## 2.2 Patients and methods

This is a descriptive, exploratory study with a quantitative, cross-sectional approach, carried out at the Renal Transplant Outpatient Clinic of the Hospital das Clínicas da UFPE, which exclusively treats patients from the Unified Health System (SUS).

The sample consisted of 122 patients. Of the transplant patients treated at the outpatient clinic, 82 were eligible. 12 died, 4 did not attend scheduled appointments during the data collection period, one (1) refused to take part and 2 dropped out of the programme, making up a group of 63 patients.

As for the pre-transplant patients, they made up a group of 59 patients and were selected for convenience, considering the data collection period and studies that assessed the occurrence of depression and/or quality of life in patients with CRF ' '(162029) . The inclusion criteria for the sample were: age over 18 and between 6 months and 2 years after transplantation. The exclusion criteria were: patients with psychiatric disorders diagnosed by the medical team. Data was collected between July and December 2007. Three data collection instruments were used (all applied by the author in a single interview): a form to characterise the sample, the Beck Depression Inventory (BDI), revised version 1979 '(1718) and the Medical Outcomes Study 36-item Short Form Health Survey (SF-36), an instrument validated in Brazil in 1997[19] .

The form used to characterise the sample includes identification and demographic data, as well as data on the disease and treatment.

The Beck Depression Inventory (BDI) is probably the most widely used self-assessment measure of depression, both in research and in clinical practice, having been translated into several languages and validated in different countries. Its reliability and validity are good and it can be used in clinical samples and in the general population[18] .

The overall assessment of the BDI is made by adding up the numbers next to the questions - given to the items selected by the patient. The score for the Beck scale is defined as: No depression = <15; Mild depression = 15-20; Mild to moderate depression = 20-30 and severe depression = 30-63[18] .

The original scale consists of 21 items, including symptoms and attitudes, whose intensity ranges from 0 to 3. The items refer to sadness, pessimism, feelings of guilt, feelings of punishment, self-deprecation, self-accusation, suicidal ideas, bouts of crying, irritability, social withdrawal, indecision, distortion of body image, inhibition to work, sleep disturbance, fatigue, loss of appetite, weight loss, somatic preoccupation and decreased libido - ^.[11]

The SF-36 questionnaire is a generic quality of life assessment tool made up of 36 items grouped into eight components: functional capacity, physical limitations, pain, general health, vitality, social aspects, emotional aspects and mental health[5] . It is one of the most widely used instruments for assessing quality of life, applicable to various types of diseases, and therefore assesses health-related quality of life \.(9

To assess the results, scores were calculated, with each answer corresponding to a specific score. This value was then transformed into scores for eight domains, ranging from 0 (zero) to 100 (one hundred), where 0 (zero) is considered the worst value and 100 (one hundred) the best for each domain \.(19

SPS 13.0 for Windows and Excel 2003 software were used to enter the data and all the tests were applied with 95% reliability.

The Kolmogorou-Smimov normality test was used for quantitative variables. The existence of association was verified using Fisher's Exact Test and the Chi-square test for categorical variables, the Mean Test; Student's T-test (normal distribution) and Mann-Whitney (non-normal); the Mean Test (with more than two groups); Anova (normal distribution) and Kruskal Wallis (non-normal) were also used to statistically analyse the data.

All the patients previously signed an informed consent form. The project was approved by the Research Ethics Committee of the Health Sciences Centre of the Federal University of Pernambuco, under CAAE-0049.0.172.000-07.

## 2.3 Results

Table 1 shows that: of the 59 pre-transplant patients, 34 (57.6%) were male, 32 (54.2%) lived in the Metropolitan Region of Recife, most of the group, 17 (28.8%) were retired and only 3 (5.1%) reported having no occupation at the time of the interview, 30 (50.8%) had completed primary school, 5 (8.5%) had higher education with post-graduate qualifications and only 3 (5.1%) were illiterate.

Of the 63 transplant patients, 35 (55.6%) were male, 32 (50.8%) lived in the Metropolitan Region of Recife, the majority of patients, 27 (42.8%) were beneficiaries and only 2 (3.2%) reported having no occupation at the time of the interview, 34 (53.9%) had completed primary school, 1 (1.6%) had higher education with postgraduate qualifications and only 1 (1.6%) was illiterate.

Socio-demographic characteristics were similar between the groups, demonstrating homogeneity in the sample studied.

**Table 1: Pre- and post-transplant kidney patients according to socio-demographic characteristics followed up at the Hospital das Clínicas outpatient clinic. Recife, 2007.**

| Variables | Groups | | | | p-value |
|---|---|---|---|---|---|
| | Post-transplant | | Pre-transplant | | |
| | n | % | n | % | |
| **Sex** | | | | | |
| Male | 35 | 55,6 | 34 | 57,6 | 0,962 * |
| Female | 28 | 44,4 | 25 | 42,4 | |
| **Residence** | | | | | |
| RMR | 32 | 50,8 | 32 | 54,2 | 0,842 * |
| Others | 31 | 49,2 | 27 | 45,8 | |
| **Occupation** | | | | | |
| Professional activity | 18 | 28,6 | 13 | 22,0 | 0,123 ** |
| Home | 6 | 9,5 | 5 | 8,5 | |
| Retired | 7 | H,1 | 17 | 28,8 | |
| Beneficiary | 27 | 42,8 | 16 | 27,1 | |
| Student | 3 | 4,8 | 5 | 8,5 | |
| No occupation | 2 | 3,2 | 3 | 5,1 | |
| **Education** | | | | | |
| Illiterate | 1 | 1,6 | 3 | 5,1 | 0,294 ** |
| Elementary school incomplete | 3 | 4,8 | 4 | 6,8 | |
| Complete primary education | 34 | 53,9 | 30 | 50,8 | |

| Completed high school | 24 | 38,1 | 17 | 28,8 |
| University degree with postgraduate qualification | 1 | 1,6 | 5 | 8,5 |

(*) Chi-Square test

(**) Fisher's Exact Test

Table 2 shows that: the average age of the pre-transplant patients was 47 ± 12.38 years, the median income was R$ 380.00 and the average time on dialysis was 39.63 months, equivalent to 3 years and 3 months.

Among the transplant recipients, the average age was 39 ± 10.39 years, income was also R$ 380.00 and the average time on dialysis was 82.05 months, equivalent to 6 years and 10 months.

The average transplant time was 1 year and 3 months. This data is not shown in the table, as it only refers to one of the groups studied; however, it is covered in the discussion.

The average dialysis time was also covered in the discussion, due to its relevance to the study.

**Table: Pre- and post-transplant kidney patients according to age, income and time on dialysis, followed up at the Hospital das Clínicas outpatient clinic. Recife, 2007**

| Variables | Groups | | | | p-value |
| | Post-transplant | | Pre-transplant | | |
| | Average | DP | Average | DP | |
| Age | 39,3 | ±10,39 | 47,1 | ±12,38 | 0,000 * |
| | Median | Q1; Q3 1 | Median | Q1;Q3 | |
| Income | 380,00 | 380,00; 900,00 | 380,00 | 380,00; 700,00 | 0,328 ** |
| | Average | DP | Average | DP | |
| Dialysis time | 6,8 | ±4,51 | 3,3 | ±2,79 | 0,000 ** |

(1) Student's t-test

(2) ) Mann-Whitney test

Table 3 shows that 47 (79.6%) patients pre-transplant had no depression, 7 (11.9%) had moderate to severe depression, 4 (6.8%) mild depression and 1 (1.7%) had severe depression.

Among the transplant recipients: 56 (88.9%) had no depression, 4 (6.3%) had moderate to severe depression, 3 (4.8%) had mild depression and no patients had severe depression.

**Table 3: Pre- and post-transplant kidney patients according to levels of depression, followed up at the Hospital das Clínicas outpatient clinic. Recife, 2007**

| Depression levels | Groups | | | | p-value * |
| | Post-transplant | | Pre-transplant | | |
| | n | % | n | % | |
| No Depression | 56 | 88,9 | 47 | 79,6 | |

| | n | % | n | % | p-value * |
|---|---|---|---|---|---|
| Mild Depression | 3 | 4,8 | 4 | 6,8 | |
| Moderate to severe depression | 4 | 6,3 | 7 | 11,9 | 0,470 |
| Severe Depression | 0 | 0,0 | 1 | 1,7 | |
| **Total** | **63** | **100,0** | **59** | **100,0** | |

(*) Fisher's Exact Test

Table 4 shows that 38 (86.4%) of the transplant recipients, who were between 1 and 2 years into their transplant, had no depression, 4 (9.1%) had moderate to severe depression and 2 (4.5%) had mild depression. Among the transplant patients who had been transplanted for 1 year or less, 18 (94.7%) had no depression and only 1 (5.3%) had mild depression.

**Table 4: Pre- and post-transplant kidney patients according to levels of depression, according to time since transplantation, followed up at the Hospital das Clínicas outpatient clinic. Recife, 2007**

| Depression levels | Transplant time | | | | p-value * |
|---|---|---|---|---|---|
| | ≤ 1 year | | > 1 year and ≤ 2 years | | |
| | n | % | n | % | |
| No Depression | 18 | 94,7 | 38 | 86,4 | |
| Mild Depression | 1 | 5,3 | 2 | 4,5 | |
| Moderate to severe depression | 0 | 0,0 | 4 | 9,1 | 0,547 |
| **Total** | **19** | **100,0** | **44** | **100,0** | |

(*) Fisher's Exact Test

Table 5 shows that among patients with less than 4 years of dialysis, 49 (83%) had no depression, 6 (10.2%) had mild depression, 3 (5.1%) moderate to severe depression and 1 (1.7%) severe depression.

Among the patients who had been on dialysis for between 4 and 8 years, 30 (90.9%) had no depression, 2 (6.1%) had moderate to severe depression, only 1 (3%) had mild depression and no patients had severe depression.

Among the patients who had been on dialysis for 8 years or more, 24 (80%) had no depression, 6 (20%) had moderate to severe depression and none of the sample had mild or severe depression.

**Table 5: Pre- and post-transplant kidney patients according to levels of depression, according to length of time on dialysis, followed up at the Hospital das Clínicas outpatient clinic. Recife, 2007**

| Depression levels | Dialysis time | | | | | | p-value* |
|---|---|---|---|---|---|---|---|
| | < 4 years | | 4 \|-8 | | ≥8 | | |
| | n | % | n | % | n | % | |
| No Depression | 49 | 83,0 | 30 | 90,9 | 24 | 80,0 | |
| Mild Depression | 6 | 10,2 | 1 | 3,0 | 0 | 0,0 | |
| Moderate to Severe Depression | 3 | 5,1 | 2 | 6,1 | 6 | 20,0 | 0,089 |
| Severe Depression | 1 | 1,7 | 0 | 0,0 | 0 | 0,0 | |
| Total | 59 | 100,0 | 33 | 100,0 | 30 | 100,0 | |

(*) Fisher's Exact Test

Table 6 shows that: in pre-transplant patients, social aspects, limitations due to emotional aspects and mental health had the highest means, corresponding to 90.0 (± 23.53 SD), 77.4 (± 41.73 SD) and 76.6 (± 19.76 SD) respectively, followed by the domains: pain, with 69.3 (± 30.20 SD), limitation by physical aspects, with 68.6 (± 45.15 SD), vitality, with 67.0 (± 22.95), functional capacity, representing 66.1 (± 31.43 SD) and, lastly, general state of health, with 63.7 (± 24.48).

Among the transplant recipients, the following domains stood out: limitation due to emotional aspects, with 87.8 (± 32.41 SD), functional capacity, with 82.6 (± 22.38 SD) and social aspects, with 82.1 (± 30.18 SD), followed by: vitality, with 80.4 (± 21.8 SD), pain, 78.8 (±

31.65 SD), mental health 74.1 (± 21.45 SD) and, lastly, general health status, with 71.1 (± 28.47 SD).

**Table 6: Pre- and post-transplant kidney patients according to mean scores in the domains of the SF-36 questionnaire, followed up at the Hospital das Clínicas outpatient clinic. Recife, 2007**

| Domains of the SF-36 | Groups | | p-value |
|---|---|---|---|
| | Post-transplant | Pre-transplant | |
| | Mean ± SD | Mean ± SD | |
| Functional Capacity | 82,6 ±22,38 | 66,1 ±31,43 | 0,001 * |
| Limitation by physical aspects | 77,0 ±41,71 | 68,6 ±45,15 | 0,335 * |
| Pain | 78,8 ±31,65 | 69,3 ± 30,20 | 0,027 * |
| General state of health | 71,1 ±28,47 | 63,7 ± 24,48 | 0,049 * |
| Vitality | 80,4 ±21,58 | 67,0 ± 22,95 | 0,000 * |
| Social Aspects | 82,1 ±30,18 | 90,0 ± 23,53 | 0,099 * |
| Limitation by Emotional Aspects | 87,8 ± 32,41 | 77,4 ±41,73 | 0,111 * |
| Mental Health | 74,1 ±21,45 | 76,6 ±19,76 | 0,502 ** |

(*) Mann-Whitney test

(**) Student's t-test

Table 7 shows that: for the group with time less than or equal to 1 year, the highest percentile corresponded to limitation due to emotional aspects, with 91.2 (± 26.86 SD), followed by: pain, with 86.0 (± 25.4 SD), functional capacity, 83.0 (± 17.58 SD), vitality, 80.79 (± 18.13 SD), limitation by physical aspects, 76.3 (± 41.23 SD), social aspects, 75.7 (± 31.86 SD), mental health, 74.5 (± 16.72 SD) and, lastly, general state of health, with 66.1 (± 30.54 SD).

The following domains were observed in decreasing order for the group with a transplant time of one year or more: limitation by emotional aspects, 86.4 (± 34.71 SD), social aspects, 84.9 (± 29.36 SD), functional capacity, 82.5 (± 24.34 SD), vitality, 80.2 (± 42.39 SD), pain, 75.8 (± 33.8 SD), mental health, 73.9 (± 23.38 SD) and, lastly, general state of health, with 73.3 (± 27.61 SD).

**Table 7: Pre- and post-transplant kidney patients according to mean scores in the domains of the SF-36 questionnaire, according to time since transplantation, followed up at the Hospital das Clínicas outpatient clinic. Recife, 2007**

| Domains of the SF-36 | Transplant time | | p-value |
| --- | --- | --- | --- |
| | ≤ 1 year | ≤ 2 years old | |
| | Mean ± SD | Mean ± SD | |
| Functional Capacity | 83,0 ± 17,58 | 82,5 ± 24,34 | 0,433 * |
| Limitation by Aspects Physical | 76,3 ±41,23 | 77,3 ± 42,39 | 0,594 * |
| Pain | 86,0 ± 25,40 | 75,8 ± 33,80 | 0,263 * |
| General state of health | 66,1 ±30,54 | 73,3 ± 27,61 | 0,442 * |
| Vitality | 80,79 ± 18,13 | 80,2 ±23,10 | 0,733 * |
| Social Aspects | 75,7 ±31,86 | 84,9 ± 29,36 | 0,187* |
| Limitation by Emotional Aspects | 91,2 ±26,86 | 86,4 ± 34,71 | 0,678 * |
| Mental Health | 74,5 ± 16,72 | 73,9 ±23,38 | 0,918 ** |

(*) Mann-Whitney test

(**) Student's t-test

Table 8 shows that: in the group with less than 4 years of dialysis, the highest averages followed one another in decreasing order: social aspects, 85.6 (± 28.13 SD), limitation by emotional aspects, 78 (± 41.8 SD), pain, 77.6 (± 29.72 SD), limitation by physical aspects, 74.6 (± 42.67 SD), mental health, 72.8 (± 29.73 SD), vitality, 71.69 (± 21.67 SD), and general state of health, 65.8 (± 25.75 SD).

In the group with dialysis time between 4 and 8 years, the highest average was in limitations due to emotional aspects, with 91.9 (± 26.39 SD), followed by social aspects, 87.9 (± 26.61 SD), mental health, 81.6 (± 16,18 dp), vitality, 78.9 (± 20.98 dp), functional capacity, 78.9 (± 25.53 dp), limitations due to physical aspects, 75 (± 43.3 dp), pain, 74.2 (± 29.5 dp) and, lastly, general state of health, 71.4 (± 27.68).

In the group with 8 or more years of dialysis, the following were observed in descending order: social aspects, 84.58 (± 27.4 SD), limitation due to emotional aspects, 82.2 (± 37.89 SD), functional capacity, 73.7 (± 28.62 SD), vitality, 72.7 (± 27.82 SD), pain, 67.5 (± 35.56 SD), limitation due to physical aspects, 67.5 (± 46.03 SD) and, lastly, general state of health, 66.6 (± 28.16 SD).

**Table 8: Pre- and post-transplant kidney patients according to mean scores on the domains of the SF-36 questionnaire, according to length of time on dialysis, followed up at the Hospital das Clínicas outpatient clinic. Recife, 2007**

| Domains of SF-36 | Dialysis time | | | p-value |
| --- | --- | --- | --- | --- |
| | < 4 years<br>Mean ± SD | 4 \|-8<br>Mean ± SD | ≥8<br>Mean ± SD | |
| Functional Capacity | 72,8 ± 29,73 | 78,8 ± 25,53 | 73,7 ± 28,62 | 0,680 * |
| Limitation by Physical Aspects | 74,6 ±42,67 | 75,0 ±43,30 | 67,5 ±46,03 | 0,642 * |
| Pain | 77,6 ±29,72 | 74,2 ± 29,50 | 67,5 ± 35,56 | 0,376 * |
| General state of Health | 65,8 ± 25,75 | 71,4 ±27,68 | 66,6 ±28,16 | 0,444 * |
| Vitality | 71,69 ±21,67 | 78,9 ± 20,98 | 72,7 ± 27,82 | 0,210 * |
| Social Aspects | 85,6 ±28,13 | 87,9 ± 26,61 | 84,58 ± 27,40 | 0,638 * |
| Limitation by Emotional Aspects | 78,0 ±41,80 | 91,9 ±26,39 | 82,2 ± 37,89 | 0,256 * |
| Mental Health | 74,4 ± 19,57 | 81,6 ±16,18 | 70,3 ± 25,38 | 0,082 ** |

(*) Kruskal-Wallis

(**) Anova

## 2.4  Discussion

The study showed that there was no statistically significant difference in depression between pre-transplant and renal transplant patients. However, there was a trend towards more cases of depression among pre-transplant patients (table 3), in line with results obtained in another study[16] . However, it should be emphasised that depression can be a potential problem post-transplant, due to some possible implications, such as lack of adherence to treatment and loss of the graft ' '[16,20,21] , as well as bodily changes, feelings of guilt towards the donor and the effect of immunosuppressants[22]

.

There was also a high percentage of patients in both groups who did not have depression (table 3). The studies carried out in this area show different results to the data found, demonstrating the presence of this disorder mainly among patients on the pre-transplant list[23] and among those transplanted who have returned to haemodialysis due to graft rejection ' ' \[13,20,21

This difference in results may be related to the fact that the study did not involve patients with rejection, which would have been expected to result in an increase in cases of depression among the subjects. We also speculate as to the repercussions of the patient's waiting time for the transplant while still on dialysis treatment, as mentioned by the authors^ ' '[242526] .

However, in the patients in whom depression was found, the pre-kidney transplant group had the highest rates of this disorder at all levels (Table 3), as reported by other authors ' ' \[202324

The causes for a higher rate of depression among patients with CRF may be related to the lifestyle acquired when they started dialysis treatment. Dietary and water restriction, loss of autonomy, a drop in monthly income, reduced sexual interest and fear of death are identified as factors causing depressive disorder in this population '[1327] . Other causes frequently related to depression in patients undergoing haemodialysis treatment are: complaints of malaise, cramps, sudden drops in blood pressure, the presence of an arteriovenous fistula and prejudice when entering the labour market[28] , as well as poor adherence to treatment .[29]

The problems experienced by patients with chronic kidney disease have a negative impact on their quality of life[5 ' ' '11233031] , 'as can be seen in table 6, where
practically all domains related to quality of life were lower compared to kidney transplant patients, as described by other authors '[2332] .

Another reason for depression in patients with CRF who are on the waiting list for a transplant is possibly the way they cope with the new situation. The stress experienced by these patients when faced with the possibility of a transplant could trigger a depressive disorder ' '[242526] .

For some patients, the waiting list for a transplant is considered a symbol of hope, of psychic and social reorganisation. For others, it can be seen as their last chance[33] .

It is worth emphasising that depression can also occur after kidney transplantation, as shown in some studies ' ' '[2130343536] 'and as observed in some patients in this study (table 3), as well as in studies of other types of transplantation, such as liver transplantation[33] , which can be explained by clinical and/or surgical complications[22] , non-adherence to treatment '[1336] , bodily changes '[2235] , the use of immunosuppressants ' '[162122 37] \ or perhaps the confluence of all these factors, in addition to negatively interfering with the QoL of these patients '[3036] \ Both depression can express the effect of one or more related factors, and it can be the cause of other problems. Untreated depression can lead to graft rejection due to non-adherence to treatment[13] , as well as being a risk factor for suicide '[3839] . Likewise, rejection can be considered a risk factor for depression and suicide^ ' -*.[1321]

With regard to the length of time since transplantation and its possible relationship with levels of depression, it was observed that the highest number of transplanted patients without depression corresponded to a period of more than one year and less than or equal to two years after the procedure. This result may be related to greater adaptation to lifestyle changes after one year of transplantation, as mentioned by the authors[40] . The patient acquires more independence[12] , due to the reduced frequency of hospital visits, has more autonomy to solve their personal problems and carry out their daily activities .[35]

Another reason would be the reduction in immunosuppressant doses, which normally occurs over time, according to the protocol of each drug, and may be related to the reduction in the effects of these medications, as is the case with depressive symptoms[37] .

However, among the transplant patients who were depressed, most were depressed during this same period, as reported in a similar study[36] \ This justifies the occurrence of depression after one year due to the financial impact related to the difficulty of reintegrating into the labour market, the physical state of the patient and the treatment they are undergoing, which influences family life and social activities, digestive changes (constipation) and worries such as fear of infection and graft rejection.

A cumulative incidence of cases of depression over three years post-transplant, however, only justifies the occurrence of this disorder in the first year, relating it to factors such as: readjustment in daily life, fear of rejection and infection, and the use of immunosuppressants, as well as their adverse effects[21] .

This study showed that the largest number of patients without depression were on dialysis for less than four years (Table 5), which differs from the findings of other studies ' ' '(1335383941) '.

This may be due to patients feeling hopeful that they will soon be able to get rid of this situation, some because of the hope they have in a possible transplant ' '(223542) , others because they don't understand what it means to have chronic kidney disease and its implications, thus thinking that there may be a cure and that the treatment is temporary[24] .

However, although the largest number of patients without depression were on dialysis for less than four years, paradoxically, the majority of those with the disorder were also on dialysis for the same period, which is in line with previously cited studies* ' ' ' ^ ).433538391

It can be inferred that this stems from the way each person copes with different situations. Each individual reacts in a certain way when surprised by the news that they have a chronic illness and will need treatment for the rest of their lives ' ^(24273) .

This can be exacerbated if the possibility of a transplant arises: the individual has often not even assimilated the illness and the treatment they will undergo, and is then faced with the prospect of surgery in which they will have to receive an organ from another person, living or dead[44] .

However, by stratifying the levels of depression in Table 5, it can be seen that there were more cases of mild depression in the period of less than four years, while most cases of moderate to severe depression were in the period of eight years or more. It is inferred that this is due to the prolonged waiting time in the pre-transplant queue, which could lead to the appearance of comorbidities[45] and even the death of the patient, as well as increasing uncertainty about the transplant being carried out, due to donor incompatibility[20] .

Table 6 shows that the kidney transplant group had a better quality of life, with a statistically significant difference in practically all the domains compared to the pre-transplant queue group, which is in line with the results of some studies ' '[23,31,32_46] , with the exception of the social aspects and mental health components, which had slightly higher percentiles among the pre-transplant queue patients.

It is inferred that the better quality of life among transplant recipients is due to the degree of independence that the transplant provides, when successful, in addition to less food restriction, absence of water restriction and greater physical well-being, as also mentioned in some studies[35_40]

.

Among the domains that stood out most in this study, when comparing the two groups, were vitality (p = 0.000), functional capacity (p = 0.001), pain (p = 0.027) and general state of health (p = 0.049). In one study[29] , there were no statistically significant differences in quality of life when comparing groups undergoing haemodialysis, peritoneal dialysis and kidney transplants. However, the vitality component was found to have a higher score in the kidney transplant group, as was found in this study.

Another study also showed no statistically significant difference between QoL scores when comparing pre- and post-kidney transplant patients; however, it did mention that the mean scores pointed to a positive difference in the assessment of quality of life after transplantation[35] .

A third study showed that subjective perception of QoL was negatively correlated with the presence of depression and lack of social support[47] .

However, despite the fact that the present study and many of the studies already mentioned show more satisfactory results in relation to QoL among kidney transplant patients, it is worth highlighting the potential impairment of QoL in the post-transplant period, in view of some concerns peculiar to this period, such as changes in body image, insecurity about a possible return to professional activities, fear of graft rejection and a return to dialysis, as corroborated by some authors ' '[7,22,32,35] ' .

With regard to the social aspect domain, the highest score was related to a small number of patients in the pre-transplant queue, who had social characteristics that were different from the others, such as higher income, better housing conditions, higher intellectual level and access to private or subsidised health treatment, which raised the average scores in this component.

As for the mental health domain, there was also a difference between the patients in the queue and the transplant patients. The fact that this domain was higher in this group did not represent statistical significance and is somewhat at odds with the data presented in table 3, which shows a higher number of cases of depression in this population, as well as a study carried out with patients undergoing dialysis treatment, in which the presence of depression was found to impair QoL, especially in the mental and physical health domains[30].

A study on predictors of quality of life in patients with chronic illness on haemodialysis found lower scores in relation to the physical and mental components, relating these results to the presence of comorbidities such as Diabetes Mellitus (DM) and Depression, the use of a CDL as a vascular access, the absence of a regular occupation and a lower level of education, which negatively influenced the QoL of this group[23]. This study found similar data for the physical limitations domain and divergent data for the mental health domain, but the results were not statistically significant.

Tables 7 and 8 show that there was no statistical significance in terms of mean QoL scores in relation to time since transplantation, according to another study[47], and time on dialysis.

With regard to transplantation, as mentioned above, a study carried out with 166 transplanted patients, 47% liver, 42.8% kidney and 10.2% heart, assessed the relationship between levels of anxiety, depression and QoL and the length of time after transplantation. Higher levels of anxiety and depression were found one year after the transplant, with negative repercussions on patients' QoL[36]. The authors justified the results as being due to concerns about the possibility of rejection, infections and future physical, social and financial well-being* \[21-25]

However, the concerns mentioned by patients are realised in all post-transplant periods and even before the transplant takes place, as they are pertinent concerns in view of the real possibility of the aforementioned alterations occurring, as mentioned in a study*[35], which reinforces the results of this study.

With regard to haemodialysis, research*[29-48] * shows that patients with a shorter period of dialysis treatment had higher QoL scores, as did patients who did not undergo dialysis treatment before transplantation. However, with regard to transplant patients who underwent dialysis before surgery, this study found no significant effects on QoL.

## 2.5 Final considerations:

The study showed that most of the domains assessed for quality of life were significantly better among transplant patients compared to patients in the pre-transplant queue. It was also found that most patients, both in the queue and post-transplant, did not suffer from depression. The length of time spent on dialysis and transplantation does not seem to interfere with patients' perception of their emotional condition and quality of life.

However, we would emphasise the importance of valuing emotional and psychosocial aspects, due to the changes that may arise both pre- and post-renal transplant.

It is believed that further research in this area is of fundamental importance in order to gain a better understanding of the management of treatment and care for chronic patients, and systematic psychological monitoring by a multi-professional team is suggested at all stages of transplantation.

## References


1    Riella MC. Principles of nephrology and hydroelectrolytic disorders. Ed. Guanabara Koogan 1996; 3(36): 475 / (48): 639-641.

2    Smeltzer SC, Bare BG. Treatise on Medical and Surgical Nursing. Guanabara 2002; 9: 1100.

3    Romão Jr JE, Chronic Kidney Disease: Definition, Epidemiology and Classification. Brazilian Journal of Nephrology 2004; V. XXVI(3).

4    D'Ávila 1996 In, Riella. Op. Cit.

5    Castro M, Caiuby AVS, Draibe SA, Canziani MEF. Quality of life of patients with chronic renal failure on haemodialysis assessed using the generic SF-36 instrument. Rev Assoe Med Bras 2003; 49:245-9.

6    Zimmermann, P. R.; Carvalho, J. O. & Mari, J. J. Impact of depression and other psychosocial factors on the prognosis of chronic renal patients. Revista de Psiquiatria do Rio Grande do Sul 2004; 26(3):312-318.

7    Bittencourt ZZLC, Alves Filho G, Mazzali M, Santos NR. Quality of life in kidney transplant patients: importance of the functioning graft. Rev. Saúde Pública 2004; 38(5): 732-734.

8    Pereira WA, Galazzi JF, Lima AS, Andrade MAC. Liver transplantation. In: Pereira WA, organiser. Manual of organ and tissue transplants. Ed. Medsi 2000; 2:203-37.

9    Butolo-Vido M.Quintella-Femandes R. Quality of life: considerations about concept and instruments of measure. Online Brazilian Journal of Nursing [serial on the Internet]. 2007 March 13; 6(2).

10   Mclntyre T, Barroso R, Lourenço M. Impact of depression on patients' quality of life. Saúde mental 2002,4(5).

11   Valderrabano F, Jofre R, Lopez-Gomez JM. Quality of life in end-stage renal disease patients. Am J Kidney Dis 2001; 38(3):443-64.

12   Castro EK. The chronic kidney patient and organ transplantation in Brazil: psychosocial aspects. *Rev. SBPH. yv^.* 2005; 8(1): 1-14.

13   Almeida AM, Meleiro AMAS. Depression and chronic renal failure. J Bras Nefrol. 2000; 22:192-200.

14   Daugirdas JT. Manual of dialysis. Ed.Medsi 2003; 3.


15   Manfro, R.C. et al. Manual of Renal Transplantation. Ed Manole 2004; 1.


16   Karaminia R, Tavallaii SA, Lorgard-Dezfuli-Nejad M, Lankarani M.M, Mirzaie HH, Einollahi B, and Firoozan A. Anxiety and Depression: A Comparison Between Renal Transplant Recipients and Hemodialysis Patients. Transplantation Proceedings 2007; 39: 1082-1084.


17   Beck, AT, Steer RA, Garbin MG. Psychometric properties of the Beck Depression Inventory: twenty-five years of evaluation. Clin. Psychol. Rev. 1988; 8(l):77-100.


18   Gorestein C, Andrade H. Beck Depression Inventory: psychometric properties of the Portuguese version. Rev Psiquiatr Clin 1998; 25:245-50.


19   Ciconelli RM. Portuguese translation and validation of the quality of life questionnaire "Medical outcomes study 36-item short form health survey (SF-36)" [thesis]. Federal University of São Paulo 1999.


20   Akman, B, Ozdemir FN, Sezer S, Micozkadioglu H, Haberal M. Depression levels before and after renal transplantation. Transplant Proc 2004; 36:111-3.


21   Dobbels F, Skeans MA, Snyder JJ, Tuomari AV, Maclean JR, and Kasiske BL. Depressive Disorder in Renal Transplantation: An Analysis of Medicare Claims. American Journal of Kidney Diseases 2008; 51 (5):819-828.


22   Abrunheiro LMM, Perdigoto R, Sendas S. Psychological Assessment and Follow-up Before and After Liver Transplantation. Psych, Health & Diseases. Nov. 2005; 6(2): 139-143.
23   Barbosa LMM, Júnior MPA, Bastos KA. Predictors of Quality of Life in Patients with Chronic Kidney Disease on Haemodialysis. J Bras Nefrol 2007; 29(4).

24   Velloso, Rosana Laura Martins. Effects of haemodialysis on the subjective field of chronic renal patients. *Cogito* 2001; 3:73-82.


25   Sasso KD, Galvão CM, Silva Jr OC, França AVC. Liver transplantation: learning outcomes for patients awaiting surgery. Rev. Latino-Am. Enfermagem 2005 Aug; 13(4):481-488.


26   Massarollo MC, Kurcgant P. The experience of nurses in the liver transplant programme of a public hospital. Rev Latino-am Enfermagem 2000; 8(4):66-72.


27   Higa K et al. Quality of life of patients with chronic renal insufficiency undergoing dyalisis treatment. Actapaul. enferm. 2008; 21.

28  Lara EA, Sarquis LMM. The chronic renal patient and their relationship with work. Cogitare Enf. 2004; 9(2):99-106.

29  Sayin A, Mutluay R, and Sindel S. Quality of Life in Hemodialysis, Peritoneal Dialysis, and Transplantation Patients. Transplantation Proceedings 2007; 39:3047-3053.

30  Noohi S, Khaghani-Zadeh M, Javadipour M, Assari S, Najafi M, Ebrahiminia M, and Pourfarziani V. Anxiety and Depression Are Correlated With Higher Morbidity After Kidney Transplantation. Transplantation Proceedings 2007; 39:1074-1078.

31  Pereira LC, Chang J, Fadil-Romão MA, Abensur H, Araújo MRT, Noronha IL, et al. Health-related quality of life in renal transplant patients. J Bras Nefrol 2003;25:10-6.

32  Overbeck, M. Bartels, O. Decker, J. Harms, J. Hauss, and J. Fangmann. Changes in Quality of Life After Renal Transplantation. Transplantation Proceedings 2005; 37:1618- 1621.

33  Duarte PM, Sankarankutty AK, Silva OC, Gorayeb R, et al. Psychic distress in patients listed for liver transplantation. Act Cir. Bras. 2006; 21(1).
34  Arapaslan B, Soykan A, Soykan C, and Kumbasar H. Cross-Sectional Assessment of Psychiatric Disorders in Renal Transplantation Patients in Turkey: A Preliminary Study. Transplantation Proceedings 2004; 36:1419-1421.

35  Ravagnani LMB, Domingos NAM, Miyazaki MCOS, Quality of life and coping strategies in patients undergoing kidney transplantation. Estudos de Psicologia. 2007; 12 (2): 177-184.

36  Pérez-San-Gregorio MA, Martín-Rodríguez A, Díaz-Domínguez R, Pérez-Bemal J. The Influence of Posttransplant Anxiety on the Long-Term Health of Patients. Transplantation Proceedings 2006; 38:2406-2408.

37  Rosenberger J, Geckova AM, Dijk JP, Roland R, Heuvel WJA, Groothof JWG Factors modifying stress from adverse effects of immunosuppressive medication in kidney transplant recipients. Clinicai Transplantation 2004; 19(1):70-76.

38  Moura Júnior JA, Souza CAM, Oliveira IR, Miranda RO, Teles C, Moura Neto JA. Suicide risk in haemodialysis patients: evolution and mortality over three years. J. bras. psiquiatr. 2008; 57(1):44-51.

39  Kurella M, Kimmel PL, f Belinda S. Young and Glenn M. Chertow. Suicide in the United States End-Stage Renal Disease Programme. J Am Soc Nephrol 2005; 16:774-781.

40  Brandão de Carvalho Lira Ana Luisa, Cavalcante Guedes Maria Vilaní, Oliveira Lopes Marcos Venícios de. Adolescent chronic kidney disease: physical, social and emotional changes after

transplantation. Rev Soc Esp Enferm Nefrol. 2005; 8(4): 12-16.

41  Almeida AM, The importance of mental health in the quality of life and survival of patients with chronic renal failure. J Bras Nefrol. 2003; 250:209-14.

42  Pietrovsk V, DalfAgnol CM. Significant situations in the space-context of haemodialysis: what do service users say? Rev. bras. enferm. [serial on the Internet]. 2006 Oct; 59(5):630-635.

43  Amato MS, Amato NV, Uip DE. Evaluation of the quality of life of patients with Chagas' disease undergoing heart transplantation. Rev. Soc. Bras. Med. Trop. 1997; 30(2): 159-160.

44  Mendes AC, Shiratori K. The perceptions of kidney transplant patients. Rev Nursing. 2002; 5 (44): 45-51.

45  Morsch C, Gonçalves L F, Barros E. Kidney disease severity index, care indicators and mortality in haemodialysis patients. Rev. Assoe. Med. Bras. 2005 Oct; 51(5):296-300.

46  Virzi A, GiammarresiSignorelli MS, Veroux MG, Maugeri S, Nicoletti A, Veroux P. Depression and Quality of Life in Living Related Renal Transplantation. Transplantation Proceedings 2007; 39 (6): 1791-1793.

47  Shah VS, Ananth A, Sohal GK, Bertges-Yost W, Eshelman A, Parasuraman RK, and Venkat KK. Quality of Life and Psychosocial Factors in Renal Transplant Recipients. Transplant Proc. 2006; 38:1283-1285.

48  Cattai GBP, Rocha FA, Nardo Júnior N., Pimentel GGA. Quality of life in patients with chronic renal failure - SF-36. Cienc Cuid Saude 2007; 6(2):460-467.

# CHAPTER 3

## APPENDICES

### A- Informed consent form

### B- Sample characterisation form

**TERM OF FREE AND INFORMED CONSENT (TCLE)**

**PROJECT**

DEPRESSION AND QUALITY OF LIFE IN PATIENTS BEFORE AND AFTER KIDNEY TRANSPLANTATION

Author's name: **Patrícia Madruga Rêgo Barros**
Name of Supervisor: **Luciane Soares de Lima**
Address: Rua Capitão Ponciano 63, Barro - Recife - PE - Zip code: 50780-040
 Contact telephone: (81) 3251.1936 e-mail: patricia-madruga@hotmail.com

The aim of the study was to analyse depression and quality of life in patients before and after kidney transplantation.

The study will be carried out at the *kidney transplant clinic of* the Hospital das Clínicas Recife - Pernambuco.

Data will be collected using a form made up of closed questions and specific inventories to analyse quality of life and depression.
This data will be used to prepare a master's thesis.
The research will be free of charge for you and you will not receive any payment for your participation.

The information obtained through the study will be kept confidential and the privacy of its participants will be respected. It may be publicised at events or in scientific publications, while preserving the identity of its participants.

The application of the data collection instrument may cause embarrassment to the patients, constituting a minimal risk for the sample, but they will be able to withdraw from the study at any time without jeopardising their care. The results of the research could help to improve the quality of care provided to the target audience, avoiding or reducing health problems.

I have read and understood the information described above and freely agree to participate in the study in question.


Recife de de.


Interviewee                                    Interviewer


Witness                                        Witness

**DATA COLLECTION FORM**

Date of collection _______//Register                              :

**IDENTIFICATION DATA**

  I.  Medical record number:_____________________

  II.  Age: _________________

  III.  Sex: 1 Male □2      Female □

  IV.  Profession: _________________

  V.  Occupation: _________________

  VI.  Education:

    1  □ Illiterate4         □ 2° grades or high school

    2  □ Literate5         □ 3° degree or higher

    3  □ 1° grade or elementary school 6 □ Postgraduate degree.

VII.  Resides: 1 □ Metropolitan region of Recife (municipality):

        2 □ Other

VIII  Monthly income:_________________________________

  IX  . Housing conditions:

    1  Has piped water and complete basic sanitation

    2  □ Has electricity

    3  □ Masonry house

    4  □ Rammed earth house

  X  . Dialysis time:_______________________________

  XI  Type of dialysis treatment at the moment:

    1  nCAPD Time: 3 □ DPI Time:

    2  □ HEMODIALYSIS Time: 4 □ DPA Time:

                5 □ Not applicable

XIL Baseline disease:

    1  □ UNDETERMINED6        □     POLYCYSTIC    KIDNEYS

    2  □ GNC7            □LES

    3  □ HAS8           □UROPATHY   +PNC

    4  □ DM9            □    OTHER

    5  □ INTERSTITIAL NEPHRITIS

XIIL Type of Transplant:

| | |
|---|---|
| 1 □ Related living donor<br>2 □ Unrelated living donor | 3 □ Cadaver donor |

XIV. Transplant time:

**ANNEXES**

**A- Research Ethics Committee approval**

39

**B- SF-36 Quality of Life Questionnaire**


**C- Beck Depression Inventory (BDI)**

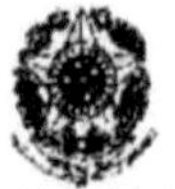



Of. N. º 007/2008 - CEP/CCS                                    Recife, 06 de outubro de 2008

Registro do SISNEP FR – 126414
CAAE – 0049.0.172.000-07
Registro CEP/CCS/UFPE Nº 051/07
**Titulo:** "**Depressão e Qualidade de Vida em Pacientes no Pré e Pós-Operatório de Transplante Renal de um Hospital Universitário de Recife-PE** "

Pesquisador Responsável: Patricia Madruga Rêgo Barros Duarte


Senhora Pesquisadora:


Informamos que o Comitê de Ética em Pesquisa envolvendo seres humanos do Centro de Ciências da Saúde da Universidade Federal de Pernambuco (CEP/CCS/UFPE) analisou e aprovou a modificação do titulo da pesquisa "**Depressão e Qualidade de Vida em Pacientes no Pré e Pós-Operatório de Transplante Renal de um Hospital Universitário de Recife-PE**".


Atenciosamente


Prof. Geraldo Bosco Lindoso Couto
Coordenador do CEP/ CCS / UFPE


A
Dra. Patricia Madruga Rêgo Barros Duarte
Programa de Pós-Graduação em Ciências da Saúde – CCS/UFPE


Av. Prof. Moraes Rego, s/n Cid. Universitária, 50670-901, Recife - PE, Tel/fax: 81 2126 8588, cepccs@ufpe.br

<table>
<tr><td colspan="2">SF-36 HEALTH RESEARCH</td><td colspan="2">SCORE</td></tr>
</table>

| Name | RG_ |
|---|---|
| Address | TEL |
| Date//      Examiner | |

**INSTRUCTIONS:** This survey asks you about your health. This information will keep us informed about *how* you feel and how well you are able to do activities of daily living. Please answer each question by marking the answer *as* indicated. If you are unsure *how to* answer, please try to answer as best you can.

1. In general, you would say that your health is:
(circle one)

    Excellent ........................................................................................1
    Very good ........................................................................................2
    Good ................................................................................................3
    Bad ..................................................................................................4
    Very bad ..........................................................................................5

2. **Compared to a year ago,** how would you rate your general health **now?**
(circle one)

    Much better now than a year ago ..................................................1
    A little better now than a year ago ...............................................2
    Almost the same as a year ago .....................................................3
    A little worse now than a year ago ...............................................4
    Much worse now than a year ago ..................................................5

3. The following items are about activities that you could currently do during an ordinary day. **Due** to **your health, do** you find it difficult to do these activities? If so, how much?

(circle a number on each side)

| Activities | Yes.<br>It's very difficult | Yes.<br>Little difficulty | No.<br>It doesn't make it any harder |
|---|---|---|---|
| A) **Vigorous activities that** require a lot of effort, such as running, lifting heavy objects, participating in strenuous sports | 1 | 2 | 3 |
| B) **Moderate activities,** such as moving a table, hoovering, playing ball, sweeping the house | 1 | 2 | 3 |
| C)**Lifting** or **carrying** supplies | 1 | 2 | 3 |
| D) Climbing **several flights of** stairs | 1 | 2 | 3 |
| E) Climb **a flight of** stairs | 1 | 2 | 3 |
| F) Bowing, kneeling or bending down | 1 | 2 | 3 |
| G) Walking **more than 1 kilometre** | 1 | 2 | 3 |
| H) Walking **several blocks** | 1 | 2 | 3 |
| I) Walk **a block** | 1 | 2 | 3 |
| J) Bathing or dressing | 1 | 2 | 3 |

4. During the **last 4 weeks,** have you had any of the following problems *with* your work or any regular daily activity **as a result of your physical health?**

(circle *a* number *in* each line)

| | Yes | No |
|---|---|---|
| A) Have you reduced **the amount of time** you dedicate to your work or other activities? | 1 | 2 |
| B) Did you do **fewer tasks** than you would have liked? | 1 | 2 |
| C) Have you been **limited in** your type of work or other activities? | 1 | 2 |
| D) Did you find it **difficult to** do your work or other activities (e.g. did you need to make *an* extra effort)? | 1 | 2 |

5. During the **last 4 weeks,** have you had any of the following problems *with* your work or other regular daily activity **as a result of an emotional problem** *(such as* feeling depressed or anxious)?

*(circle a number in each line)*

|  | Yes | No |
|---|---|---|
| A) Have you reduced the **amount of time** you dedicate to your work or other activities? | 1 | 2 |
| B) Did you do **fewer tasks** than you would have liked? | 1 | 2 |
| C) Did you not work or do any of the activities *as* **carefully as** you usually do? | 1 | 2 |

6. Over the last 4 weeks, how have your physical health or emotional problems interfered **with** your normal social activities, with family, neighbours, friends or in groups?

(circle one)

Not at all ............................................................................1
Slightly ................................................................................2
Moderately ..........................................................................3
Quite ....................................................................................4
Extremely ............................................................................5

7. How much **body pain** have you had in the **last 4 weeks?**

(circle one)

None .....................................................................................1
Very light .............................................................................2
.....................................................................................Light3
Moderate ..............................................................................4
.....................................................................................Grave5
Muitograve ..........................................................................6

8. during the **last 4 weeks,** how much has the pain interfered *with* your normal work (including both outside and inside work)?

(circle one)

.............................................................................Not at all1
A ..............................................................................little2
.........................................................................Moderately3
..........................................................................Quite a lot4
..........................................................................Exfre^mente5

9. These questions are about *how* you feel and *how* everything has been going *for you over* the **last *4* weeks.** For each question, please give an answer that comes closest to the *way* you feel.

*(circle a number for each line)*

|  | All the time | Most of the time | A good part of the time | Some of the time | A small part of the time | Nwica |
|---|---|---|---|---|---|---|
| A) How long have you felt full of vigour, full of will, full of strength? | 1 | 2 | 3 | 4 | 5 | 6 |

| | | | | | |
|---|---|---|---|---|---|
| **B)** How long have you been feeling very nervous? | 1 | 2 | 3 | 4 | 5 | 6 |
| **C)** How long have you felt so depressed that nothing could cheer you up? | 1 | 2 | 3 | **4** | 5 | 6 |
| **D)** How long have you felt calm or peaceful? | 1 | 2 | 3 | 4 | 5 | 6 |
| **E)** How long *have* you felt energised? | 1 | 2 | 3 | **4** | 5 | 6 |
| **F)** How long have you felt discouraged and down? | 1 | 2 | 3 | 4 | 5 | 6 |
| **G)** How long have you felt exhausted? | 1 | 2 | 3 | 4 | 5 | 6 |
| **H)** How long have you felt like a happy person? | 1 | 2 | 3 | **4** | 5 | 6 |
| **I)** How long have you been feeling tired? | 1 | 2 | 3 | 4 | 5 | 6 |

10.   During the last 4 weeks, how much of your time did your physical health or emotional problems interfere with your social activities (such as visiting friends, relatives, etc.)?

(circle mm)

All the ...................................................................... time 1
Most of the time ............................................................ 2
Some of the ................................................................... time 3
A small part of the ......................................................... time 4
No part of the ................................................................ time 5

11.   0 how true or false **is** each of the statements for you?

| | Definitely true | Most of the time true | I don't know | Most of the time false | Definitely wings |
|---|---|---|---|---|---|
| A) I tend to get ill a little more easily than other people | 1 | 2 | 3 | 4 | 5 |
| B) I'm as healthy as anyone I know | 1 | 2 | 3 | 4 | 5 |
| C) I think health is going to get worse | 1 | 2 | 3 | 4 | 5 |
| D) My health **is** excellent | 1 | 2 | 3 | 4 | 5 |

## SF-36 SCORING GUIDELINES

| Question | Score |
|---|---|
| 01 | 1=>5.02=>4.43=>3.44=>2.      05 =>1.0 |
| 03 | Sum nonml |
| 04 | SomaNornal |
| 05 | SomaNornal |
| 06 | 1=>52=>43=>34=>25=>1 |
| 07 | 1=>6.02=>5.43=>4.24=>3.15=>2.26=>1.0 |
| 08 | If 8=>1and 7=>1=======>6          1=>6.0<br>If 8=>1and 7->2 to 6=====>52=>4          .75<br>If 8=>2and 7=>2 to 6=====>43=>3          .75If          question 07 does not<br>If 8=>3e7=>2a6=====>34=>2.,25is          answered<br>If 8=>4e7=>2 to 6=====>25=>1.0<br>If 8=>5and 7=>2 to 6=====>1 |
| 09 | A, D, E, H = contour values (1=6, 2=5, 3=4,4=3, 5=2, 6=1)<br><br>Vitality = A + E + G + I<br><br>Mental Health = B + C + D + F + H |
| 10 | SumNominal |
| 11 | Sum of: |

| Item | Question | Limits | Score Range |
|---|---|---|---|
| A + C (nominal values)<br>B + D (contour values: 1=5, 2=4, 3=3, 4=2, 5=1) | | | |

| Item | Question | Limits | Score Range |
|---|---|---|---|
| **Functional Capacity** | 3 | 10,30 | 20 |
| **Physical Aspect** | 4 | 4,8 | 4 |
| **Pain** | 7 + 8 | 2,12 | 10 |
| **General state of health** | 1 + 11 | 5,25 | 20 |
| **Vitality** | **9 A, E, G, I** | 4,24 | 20 |
| **Social Aspects** | 6 + 10 | 2,10 | 8 |
| **Emotional Aspect** | 5 | 3,6 | 3 |
| **Mental Health** | **9 B, C, D, F, H** | 5,30 | 25 |

**Row Scale:**

$$\text{Ex: Item} = \frac{[\text{Obtained value - Lowest value}] \times 100}{\text{Variation}}$$

**Ex: Functional Capacity $=$ 21**

**Lowest value $=$ 10**

**Variation $=$ 20**

$$\frac{21 - 10}{20} \times 100 = 55$$

**Lost data:**
**If you answer more than 50% = replace with the average 0 = worst score 100 = best score**

CICONELLI, R.M.- Translation into Portuguese and Validation of the Generic Quality of Life Questionnaire "Medical Outcomes Study 36- Item Short Form Health Survey (SF-36)". Doctoral Thesis, Federal University of São Paulo, 143 pages, 1997.

## Beck Depression Inventory (BDI)

**This questionnaire consists of 21 groups of statements. After carefully reading each group, circle the number (0, 1, 2 or 3) in front of the statement in each group that best describes the way you've been feeling this week, including today. If several statements in a group seem to apply equally well, circle each one. Take care to read all the affirmations in each group before making your choice.**

**1.**0 I don't feel sad.
  1  I feel sad.
  2  I'm always sad and I can't get out of it.
  3  I'm so sad or unhappy that I can't stand it.

**2.**0 I'm not particularly despondent about the future.
  1  I feel despondent about the future.
  2  I don't think I have anything to look forward to.

3 I find the future hopeless and have the impression that things can't get any better.

**3.**0 I don't feel like a failure.
   1  I think I failed more than the average person.
   2  When I look back on my life, all I can see is a lot of failures.
   3  I think I'm a complete failure as a person.

**4.**0 I enjoy everything as much as before.
   1  I don't enjoy things as much as I used to.
   2  I find no real pleasure in anything else.
   3  I'm dissatisfied or bored with everything.

**5.**0 I don't feel particularly guilty.
   1  I feel guilty sometimes.
   2  I feel guilty most of the time.
   3  I always feel guilty.

**6.**0 I don't think he's being punished.
   1  I think I could be punished.
   2  I think I'm going to be punished.
   3  I think I'm being punished.

**7.**0 I don't feel disappointed in myself.
   1  I'm disappointed in myself.
   2  I'm disgusted with myself.
   3  I hate myself.

**8.**   0 I don't feel any worse than anyone else.
   1  I'm critical of myself because of my weaknesses or mistakes.
   2  I always blame myself for my faults.
   3  I blame myself for everything bad that happens.

**9.**0 I don't have any thoughts of killing myself.
   1  I have ideas about killing myself, but I wouldn't do it.
   2  I'd like to kill myself.
   3  I'd kill myself if I had the chance.

**10.**   0 I don't cry more than usual.
   1  I cry more now than I used to.
   2  Now I cry all the time.
   3  I used to be able to cry, but now I can't even if I want to.

**11.**0 I'm no more angry now than I ever was.
   1  I get annoyed or irritated more easily than I used to.
   2  These days I feel irritable all the time.
   3  I absolutely don't get annoyed by things that used to annoy me.

**12.**0 I haven't lost interest in other people.
   1  I'm less interested in other people than I used to be.
   2  I lost most of my interest in other people.
   3  I lost all interest in other people.

**13.**0 I make decisions more or less as well as I used to.

1  I postpone my decisions more than I used to.
2  I find it harder to make decisions than before.
3  I can't make decisions anymore.

**14.**0 I don't feel that I look any worse than I used to.
1  I worry about looking old or unattractive.
2  I feel that there are permanent changes in my appearance that make me look unattractive.
3  I consider myself ugly.

**15.**0 I can work more or less as well as before.
1  I need to make an extra effort to start anything.
2  I have to work hard to do anything.
3  I can't do any work.

**16.** 0 I sleep as well as usual.
1  I don't sleep as well as I used to.
2  I wake up an hour or two earlier than usual and have trouble getting back to sleep.
3  I wake up several hours earlier than I used to and find it hard to get back to sleep.

**17.**0 I don't get more tired than usual.
1  I get tired more easily than I used to.
2  I feel tired doing almost anything.
3  I'm too tired to do anything.

**18.**0 My appetite is no worse than usual.
1  My appetite isn't as good as it used to be.

2  My appetite is much worse now.
3  I no longer have any appetite.

**19.**0 I haven't lost much weight, if any lately.
1  I lost more than 2.5kg.
2  I lost more than 5.0kg.
3  I lost more than 7.5kg.

I'm deliberately trying to lose weight by eating less: YES () NO ()

**20.**0 I don't worry about my health any more than usual.
1  I worry about physical problems like aches and pains or stomach upsets or constipation.
2  I'm very worried about physical problems and it's hard to think about anything other than that.
3  I'm so preoccupied with my physical problems that I can't think about anything else.

**21.**0 I haven't noticed any recent changes in my sexual interest.
1  I'm less interested in sex than I used to be.
2  I'm much less interested in sex these days.
3  I completely lost interest in sex.

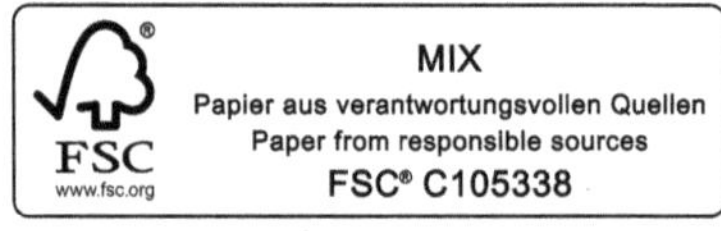

Printed by Books on Demand GmbH, Norderstedt / Germany